DEDICATION

This book is dedicated to Manny – the love of my life.

TABLE OF CONTENTS

Chapter 1- The Essentials of Weight Loss.. 5

Chapter 2- The Quickest Way to Getting Lean 11

Chapter 3- Which Diets Work Best?..17

Chapter 4- How to Manage Your Weight...21

Chapter 5-The Role of Motivation and Emotions in Weight Loss
....26

Chapter 6- Why You Should Not Skip Exercise.............................31

Chapter 7- The Basics of Weight Maintenance 37

Chapter 8- Of Pills and Surgeries..44

Chapter 9- 10 Super Foods to Muscle Building.............................48

About The Author..52

Drop Those Fats, Tone Those Muscles

Top Tricks and Tips to Losing Weight and Building Muscles

By: Kimberly Jackson

9781635014914

PUBLISHERS NOTES

Disclaimer – Speedy Publishing LLC

This publication is intended to provide helpful and informative material. It is not intended to diagnose, treat, cure, or prevent any health problem or condition, nor is intended to replace the advice of a physician. No action should be taken solely on the contents of this book. Always consult your physician or qualified health-care professional on any matters regarding your health and before adopting any suggestions in this book or drawing inferences from it.

The author and publisher specifically disclaim all responsibility for any liability, loss or risk, personal or otherwise, which is incurred as a consequence, directly or indirectly, from the use or application of any contents of this book.

Any and all product names referenced within this book are the trademarks of their respective owners. None of these owners have sponsored, authorized, endorsed, or approved this book.

Always read all information provided by the manufacturers' product labels before using their products. The author and publisher are not responsible for claims made by manufacturers.

This book was originally printed before 2014. This is an adapted reprint by Speedy Publishing LLC with newly updated content designed to help readers with much more accurate and timely information and data.

Speedy Publishing LLC

40 E Main Street, Newark, Delaware, 19711

Contact Us: 1-888-248-4521

Website: http://www.speedypublishing.co

REPRINTED Paperback Edition: 9781635014914:

Manufactured in the United States of America

Chapter 1 - The Essentials of Weight Loss

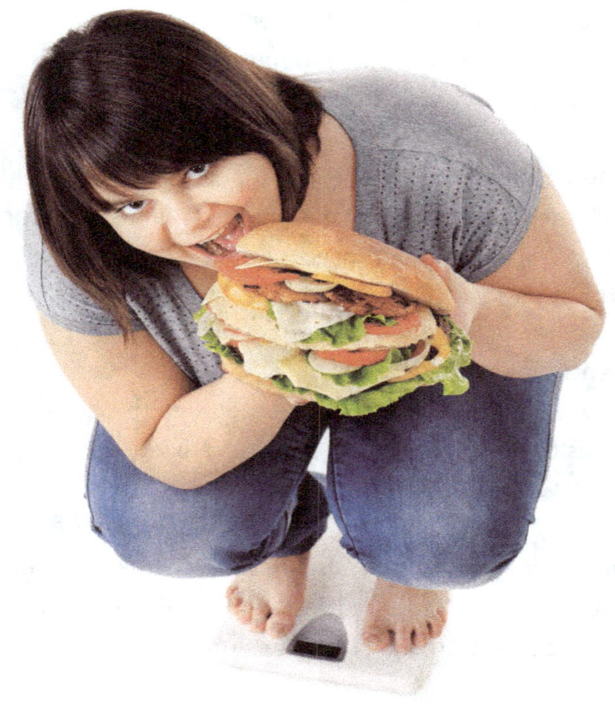

Weight loss requires a reduction in calorie consumption. Most people try to reduce weight through exercising or dieting.

Whether you want to stay fit, switch your body into a perfect one or appear sexier, you have to understand the entire concept of weight loss. If you regularly read health news, you probably recognize that the rate of obesity tends to increase. This alarming condition has awakened health practitioners and organizations. As a result, they are providing adequate tips and solutions to solve this issue. However, the help of these health agencies is not enough.

Drop Those Fats, Tone Those Muscles

If you really want to reduce your weight, you have to help yourself. You have to be more conscious with your daily lifestyle and activities.

Weight loss refers to a reduction of the total body mass characterized by a loss of skeletal muscle and body fats. This term comes in two types:

- **Intentional Weight Loss** – When a person intentionally reduces weight, they often plan a dietary or training program. These programs are designed to lose a certain amount of weight within a short period of time.

- **Unintentional Weight Loss** - Weight loss may be accidental if a person is suffering from any untreated health issues. The typical examples of these are diabetes, stress, anxiety and a lot more.

As experts claim, losing weight offers multiple benefits. Aside from a stunning appearance, you also have a chance to live for more years. Obese people often suffer from multiple diseases such as diabetes, hypertension, heart disease and cancer.

Weight Loss Considerations and Tips

Even if you opt to shed extra pounds instantly, it is still essential to avoid crash diets, fad diets, frequent fasting and other intense weight loss measures. These schemes can put you at risk for health problems.

Say for instance, people who use laxatives while dieting may develop dehydration, kidney problems, heart issues and intestinal damage.

The best way to lose more weight is to make a diet that covers adequate healthy foods. This can help in maintaining body function while shedding pounds of weight. Before doing any activities or engaging with any program, make sure that you consult with your nutritionist or doctor.

While making a weight loss plan, you should always include proper exercise. Aside from burning calories through intense physical activity, regular training develops a resting metabolism. Therefore, it can help the body to burn more calories while performing ordinary activities.

Don't Starve Yourself to Shed Off a Few Pounds

Trying to lose weight can be tough. Trying to lose weight fast can be even more of a challenge. If you think you have to starve yourself or endlessly exercise you'll be happy to learn that's not so.

Preparing for your weight loss program can make a huge difference in your success. When you take the time to evaluate your weight loss needs you'll be able to better chose the best diet and exercise program for you. Your metabolism is key to your weight loss, which is why you need to discover how fast your metabolism is. There are plenty of free metabolism calculators you can use.

What many don't realize is that to enjoy the maximum weight loss two 15 minute cardio workouts 3 to 4 times a week, combined with some weight training or resistant training on 2 to 3 times a week will result in maximizing your weight loss. The best fast weight loss combines exercise with reduced calorie intake. It will provide you with the quickest results. As you build muscle, you'll it takes more calories to maintain that muscle and so you'll lose more fat.

Drop Those Fats, Tone Those Muscles
Don't waste your time with crunches. All you'll do is develop muscle under the fat and you'll actually look fatter. Cardio workouts are ten times more effective so take advantage of them. There's no need to have to spend any money to enjoy your cardiac workout other than a pair of comfortable shoes. Walking briskly is an excellent cardio workout. Of course, you can add cycling, jogging, running, or other activities, which you enjoy.

The best diet is a healthy diet. That means avoiding processed foods and eating plenty of fresh fruits and vegetables, as well as quality protein (poultry and fish) and complex carbs. Then all you need to do is take in fewer calories than you use.

You can do this by either eating less or by exercising more. There's really no big secret here. If you reduce your calorie intake start with a 100 to 200 calorie reduction. Never drop more than 500 calories or you risk scaring your body into starvation mode because when that happens you'll not lose a pound.

To learn you can lose weight quickly is rather exciting. It's great to discover it doesn't have to take months to lose those pounds. In fact, you can easily lose 3 to 5 pounds a week and you can do it without any risk to your health. In no time, at all you'll be leaner, thinner, and more toned.

Listen to the Experts

Weight gain is frustrating when you're trying everything you can think of to shed those pounds. You watch what you eat, you exercise, and still...the pounds stay. Everyone knows that eating too much, eating fried or fatty foods, eating sugary foods, drinking alcohol and soda can lead to excess weight gain, but even those who avoid all these things find themselves putting on the pounds.

So how can you lose weight fast in a healthy manner? The good news is it isn't as difficult as you might have thought. According to some experts, a few key techniques can help you quickly shed those extra pounds. Losing weight quickly requires more than eating less and exercising more. To lose weight fast you need to combine exercise, diet, dietary supplements, and emotional support. Here are a few more techniques to help you lose weight:

* Listen to your body – Adjust your exercise and your diet to correspond with your goals and your body.

* Set goals that are realistic – Make sure you set goals that can be achieved; stay motivated, and stay focused.

* Drink more water – Drinking water removes toxins from the body. It also keeps you feeling full.

* Eat more fiber – Fiber help to fill you faster and you stay feeling full for longer.

* Remain consistent – Your success depends on remaining consistent with your plan.

* Stay away from packaged and processed foods – these foods have little nutrition, too much fat, too much sodium, and they are just plain bad for you and your waistline.

There are all kinds of diet supplements on the market. Some may be helpful, some are of no value, and some are dangerous. Before you take any diet supplements make sure you do your homework and understand how and if they can help. Quick weight loss can occur without the use of supplements.

Drop Those Fats, Tone Those Muscles
If you've ever watched "The Biggest Loser," you'll know that you can safely lose significant weight in one month if you want to. It's important to realize that losing weight involves more than just losing fat. Weight loss involves the body's water, muscle tissue, and bone mass.

Rapid weight loss can entail dehydration, loose skin, cramping, diarrhea, and fatigue. So while you can safely lose weight quickly, you can only do this providing you understand your nutritional needs vs. your weight loss, and what your limits are. You should also never undertake a weight loss program without first discussing it with your physician.

Chapter 2- The Quickest Way to Getting Lean

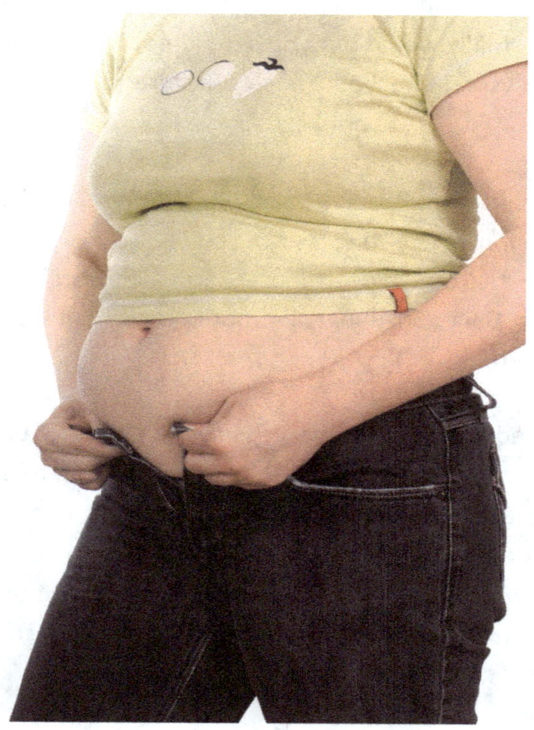

You'll be happy to know that there's no reason you can't build muscle and lose fat fast. Once you've turned fat into muscle, with a few changes to lifestyle you can look lean and fit for the rest of your life. But how does one get started in building muscle and losing fat? Glad you asked! And there's great news because you can do it quickly.

The quickest way to build your muscle mass is to get stronger. Any type of strength training will work. There's weight training that involves dumbbells, barbells, and exercises like squats. You can use either free weights or weight machines.

Drop Those Fats, Tone Those Muscles

As you build muscle, your body fat will decrease. Along with strength training, you need 30 minutes of cardio exercise three times a week. The goal here is not to exhaust yourself but rather to burn fat. When doing your cardio you should be breathing heavier than you normally would but you should not be gasping for air. You should always talk to your doctor before starting any exercise program.

You can't build your muscles unless you are feeding them properly, and when you are eating right, you'll also be losing fat. Your nutrition needs to include at least 1 gram of protein per pound of body weight daily. So things like poultry, fish, and eggs are good sources of protein.

You also need the good fats, which include omega 3, 6, and 9 found in things like olive oil and fish oil. Make sure you are eating plenty of veggies, especially the greens. Steam don't cook. All kinds of fruit are good for you, and you'll also want to make sure your eating only whole grain foods. Water is critical to your fast fat loss program. Stay away from packaged foods and fast foods, and get rid of the soda.

As well as eating healthy, you are going to have to reduce your calorie intake. Don't do anything drastic because that triggers the body to think it's in starvation mode and it actually becomes more difficult to lose those pounds. Instead, reduce gradually. The first week cut out 500kcal. After a week check to see if you've lost weight and reduce more as necessary. Never cut more calories if you see you are losing weight.

Keeping a journal can help to motivate you and stay on track. There are even free websites that allow you to track your progress online.

The Secrets behind Quick Weight Loss without the Lose Skin

Weight loss – there's a lot of buzz around it, but how do you lose weight and build muscle fast? Glad you asked! It's time the secret was out.

The weight loss industry is a multibillion dollar industry and they'd like everyone to believe there's some big secret that they know and you don't. That's how they sell you magic weight loss formulas. It's time you knew the truth about what it takes to lose weight and build muscle fast.

Muscle vs. Fat

If you are trying to lose weight and build muscle and you want to do it fast, crash diets that seriously restrict your caloric intake aren't what you need. When you lose weight while dieting, you lose muscle and fat. Exercise will preserve your muscle and build new muscle. You need to eat healthy and incorporate a vigorous exercise regime into your daily life. That will build muscle and you can watch the fat shrink away.

The Right Foods to Build Your Muscles

If you want to build your muscles, you are going to have to feed them, and not just any food – the right foods. Proteins are key to building your muscles. This is why bodybuilders use protein shakes to bulk up. But don't ignore carbs, because they are also important to building muscles.

The key to losing weight and building muscles quickly is to eat a balanced diet. You should be taking in two grams of protein per kilogram of body weight if you are following a serious exercise regime, however if you are not exercising you should be taking in no more than .8 grams per kilogram of body weight.

Calorie Counting

Without ever cutting calories, increasing your exercise and you can see an amazing reduction in weight loss. The formula to weight loss is really no secret. You must use more calories than you take in. So start paying attention and make sure you are burning up more than you are taking in. You also need to make better food choices — healthier choices mean you'll have more energy and feel fuller.

Building Muscle

You aren't going to bulk up overnight. If that's your goal and you put the time in you'll see the result in a few weeks, without any magic potions or pills. Start slow, with weights you are comfortable working with. Always do your exercises properly. Match your goals and your training to get the results you expect.

There you have it. There's really no big secret. The right mix of diet and exercise and you'll be toned and lighter in no time at all. You really can lose weight and build muscle fast.

Tips to Muscle Building

If you want to build muscle and lose body fat these three tips can accomplish both. After all, you want to lose weight (body fat) without sacrificing muscle. Good news — this can be done you properly tackle the challenge. However, to gain muscle while losing weight you really have to have your nutrition and exercise program right on the money.

You also have to understand that muscle weights more than fat. Therefore, as you build more muscle your weight may actually go up while you find your waist size going down. In the last decade, there have been significant advancements in the nutritional advances, which is why today's bodybuilder can stay lean and muscular twelve months of the year. It's all about your calorie intake vs. your calorie burn.

It's about balance. You need to take in enough calories to lose weight and gain muscle but not so many calories that you gain fat. You also need to find the right workout balance. Go for a lower number of sets and reps using a heavier weight. You should train each muscle group only one every week. On top of weight training your cardio workout is important. It needs to be intense and short.

The best 3 tips to build muscle and lose body fat are:

1. Figure out how many calories you use a day and then make sure you are not taking in more calories than that.

2. Ensure your weight training is heavy so that it will stimulate muscle growth. If you don't use heavy weights you won't stimulate the growth you desire. Weight training can be accomplished with a set of free weights. Dumbbells can be purchased cheap, and you can even get creative and use cans. Squats, lunges, and sit-ups are a good weight training exercises that cost you nothing.

3. Make sure your cardio workout is short and intense. It's a common misconception that the longer cardio sessions do a better job of burning fat and preserving the lean muscle mass.

Losing weight and developing muscles can be done quickly and efficiently without jeopardizing your health. While there are all kinds of supplements on the market promoting fast weight loss. Far too many of these supplements are all hype and no substance. Many others are little more than vitamins. Before you spend your money, it pays to do your homework.

CHAPTER 3- WHICH DIETS WORK BEST?

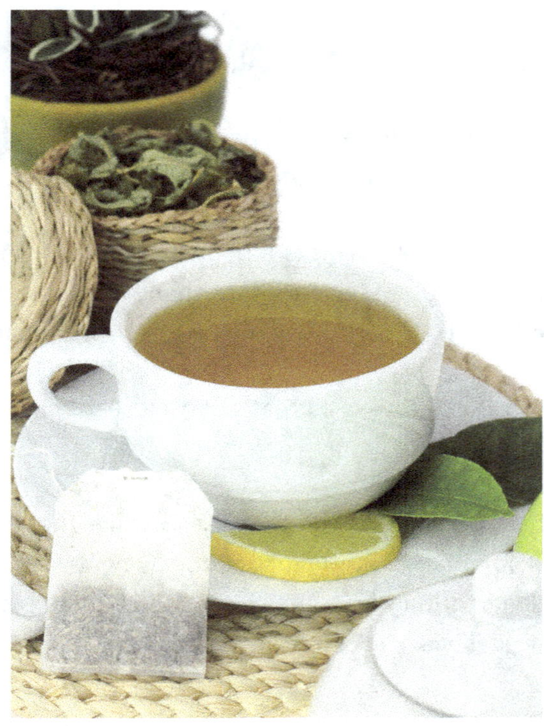

For most of us those pounds go on faster than they come off. But which diets are best to lose weight fast? Glad you asked! When it comes to fast weight loss some diets work better than others, and regardless of your diet choice it's important to add an exercise component too.

It's also important to choose a diet that you can stick to. There's no point in choosing a diet considered a fast weight loss program if you can't stand the foods that are in it.

Let's look at some of your diet options others have found useful to lose weight fast:

Scarsdale Diet – This is a diet known for its choices, which makes it easier to stick to. It's also a good choice if you're the type of person that doesn't want to be going around hungry. There's no weighting, counting, or measuring. Just follow the simple menus.

The Lemonade Diet – If you're a person with a strong willpower you might consider this combination cleanse diet.

The Cabbage Soup Diet – This is a popular choice for anyone who doesn't want to be on a diet for more than seven days. It's cheap and it's repetitive. It works but you had better like cabbage.

The Three Day Diet – This is a great way to lose 10 pounds in three days.

What one has to remember is that these while these diets have worked well for many who want to lose weight fast, they don't necessarily lead to long term weight loss if they aren't combined with healthy lifestyle choice. That includes nutritious eating and exercise.

Your exercise program doesn't have to be costly or difficult. A brisk walk that gets your heart rate up and some weight training right in your living room will do the trick. Resistance exercises are great for toning muscles, as are squats, pushups, and lunges. You might want to add a set of dumbbells to the mix but you can also use cans. Be creative. Of course, for some the gym membership is a way to keep them focused and on track. Whatever works for you. That's what's important.

While diets may start to see the pounds melt away fast, you need to make healthy food choices to enjoy the long term benefits. That includes eating fresh veggies and fruits, good protein such as poultry and fish, and avoiding packaged and processed foods.

With just a little effort you can look and feel better in no time at all. Watch those pounds melt away.

The Benefits of Fad Diets

Some people believe that fad diets are quite detrimental to their health. However, this is not always the case. It is merely how you pick the best fad diet available in the market. If you are planning to practice any fad diet, expect that you will get the succeeding benefits:

- Motivation – The ultimate challenge of losing weight is to stay motivated. If you change your exercise and eating habits, it needs a major commitment. Sometimes, when you have noticed that the results are too slow, you may feel discouraged or frustrated. However, if you continue the process, you will notice that you are reducing more fat and have the perfect body you desired to get.

- Offers Good Health – Fad diets like raw diets eliminate all foods that are processed or cooked. They also focus on consuming fresh vegetables and fruits. The Atkins diet, on the other hand, helps in reducing the intake of carbohydrates. The ultimate key to achieving good health is through consuming various foods that are rich in vitamins and nutrients.

- Awareness – A fad diet may leave you feeling active or energized. Whatever type of fad diet you opt to practice, you should always be conscious of the different foods that you need to eat. You will also know which foods are perfect for your body condition and which are not.

With great information about these fad diets, you can easily decide which of them fit the needs of your healthy body condition. After finding the best diets, make sure that you follow each step and be conscious with your daily lifestyle activities.

CHAPTER 4- HOW TO MANAGE YOUR WEIGHT

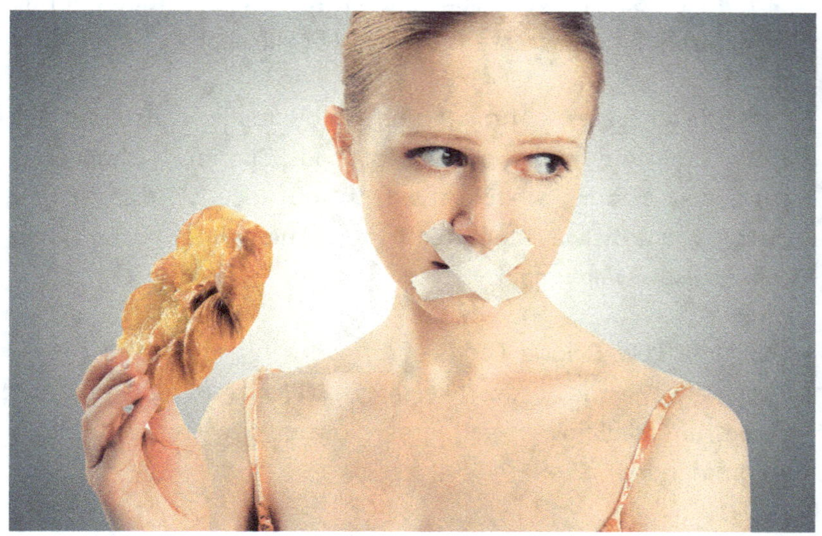

Weight management is defined as an enduring approach to a healthy lifestyle. It covers a balance of physical exercise and healthy eating to link energy intake and energy expenditure. Understanding the needs of your body is essential to weight management. It can also control over and under consumption of foods.

Nutritionists claim that weight management does not cover fad diets. It often focuses on the long-term outcomes followed by body weight maintenance. If you manage your weight, you can achieve not only a perfect figure, but prevent chronic diseases as well.

Methods of Weight Management

Weight management comes in multiple methods. Some are easy to follow while others need constant monitoring and strict implementation. To get more details about these schemes, here are some of its various methods you should know:

- More Protein Intake – Food specialists claim that protein intake at breakfast has higher effect compared to succeeding meals. It also consists of a greater thermogenic effect than fats and carbohydrates. If you consume high protein food during breakfast, it helps increase the activity of glucagon.

- Use Smaller Plates – Through the use of smaller plates, it helps you to consume smaller portions of foods. Therefore, chances to eat fewer calories are observed. If you keep on using larger plates, you are always tempted to consume greater portions and that leads to weight gain.

- Consume Low Calorie Foods – An average decrease in calorie intake always lead to slow weight loss. Picking lettuce, broccoli, grapefruit, cauliflower and other low calorie foods is highly recommended.

- Eating More Dairy Foods – Most nutritionists claim that consuming dairy foods can reduce body fat. It happens because a greater amount of dietary calcium develops the amount of energy and fat removed from the body.

- Give Up Soda or Sugary Drinks – One of the main contributors in weight gain is sugary drinks. Even if these drinks are delicious and appear harmless, carbonated drinks consist of a large amount of calories. To avoid calories, you should always drink more water. Experts suggest the consumption of eight to ten glasses of water regularly.

- Get Adequate Sleep – Since most people are busy doing their personal activities, they often neglect to practice proper sleeping habits. If you sleep on time, it helps to increase the metabolism and relieves the body of stress. These aspects are connected to weight loss and rapid metabolism.

With your understanding about these schemes, you can do the methods that will help to reduce fat and maintain a healthy lifestyle.

The Benefits of Losing and Managing Weight

Do you have an excess in body fat? If yes, then, you probably have your own reason why you opt to burn more fat and achieve a perfect body weight condition. Why do people prefer to lose weight? An ideal body figure and weight condition offers multiple benefits.

If you are not familiar with these benefits, here they are:

- Appear Sexy and Attractive – If you keep on asking why most people prefer to lose weight, most of them give similar answers. Both men and women wish to reduce more body fat to make them sexier.

- Look Healthier and Active – If you are planning to lose weight, you need to eat nutritious foods like fruits and vegetables. As a result, you will achieve a perfect body figure while getting the benefit of practicing a healthy lifestyle.

- Saves More Money – When you are losing weight, you need to consume healthy foods. Therefore, you don't need to buy any food that can destroy your eating habits. This can help you by saving you more cash.

- Know How to handle Your Health Condition – If you wish to lose weight, you should probably start by consulting your doctor. Through this, you will learn several things about how to lose weight and how to live healthy.

Drop Those Fats, Tone Those Muscles

With the various benefits of weight loss, everyone is encouraged to deal with reliable dietary and training programs. Like others, you don't need to rely on multiple programs. Though you keep on entering in several activities, it will never be effective if you don't have self-control or motivation. So, make sure that you always follow your schedule to ensure effective results.

Weight loss management is not too complicated. If you have a specific goal, all you need to do is to find ways of how to achieve it. Through the help of weight loss management, you are guided to the specific activities you need to do. You will also know the different foods that you need to eat.

For beginners, they may find it hard to follow their schedules. However, if they are eager to reach their goal, everything will turn out to be fine. This is the reason why most people prefer to lose weight using a special management program.

Are you worried about your excessive fat? If yes, then, you don't need to suffer from its consequences. Don't allow other people to bully you just because your physical appearance. If you are obese, then, you need to find ways to solve this at hand. Through practicing a weight loss plan and management, everything will be in good condition. After several weeks and months, you will realize that you are losing more fat.

Whether you want to lose weight or just want to maintain a healthy body figure, there is always a specific way of how to achieve that goal. After burning fatter, you are confident to face other people. You are also free to wear any apparel you like.

Through following these different guides, you are free to do everything you want. So, start changing your daily activity now!

Kimberly Jackson
Learn how to practice a healthy lifestyle and see how it affects your weight condition.

CHAPTER 5-THE ROLE OF MOTIVATION AND EMOTIONS IN WEIGHT LOSS

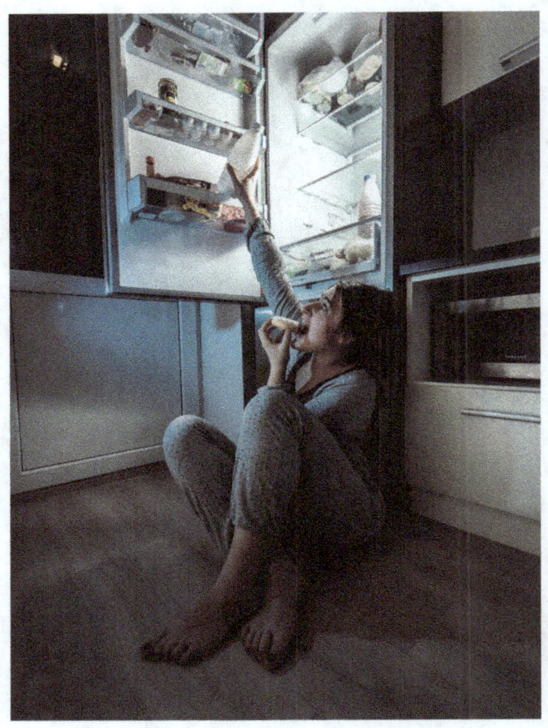

If you find yourself needing to lose weight, you're not alone. But saying you want to lose weight and actually watching those pounds disappear are two different things. Let's be honest – we're creatures of habit and we don't make change easy. That's why you want to use these 10 ways to motivate yourself to lose weight fast.

1. Play the If I Do vs. the If I Don't Game

Grab a piece of paper. Draw a line down the middle and one side write "If I Do" and on the other side write, "If I don't." You're looking into the future now. What will your life be like a month, a year, five years from now if you take action and lose the weight or if you don't take action and lose the weight? Be honest with yourself.

For example, if I do lose the weight in one year I'll be able to eat what I want without worrying about getting fat. Or If I don't lose the weight in five years, I'm likely to be diabetic. This is a great exercise for motivating yourself – just be real!

2. Don't Let Anything Get in Your Way

If you have decided to lose the weight and look great don't let anything get in your way. You can achieve your goal when you set your mind to it but you need to have a plan. For example, you decide you are going to exercise 30 minutes on the stationary bike while watching your favorite television show. Or perhaps you've decided you are going to go f a 15 minute walk after work every day. Don't let excuses stop you from doing what you have set out to do. It's really easy to say put it off. I'm tired, I have company, and I have to do laundry. Stick to your guns and you'll see the pounds start to roll off. It's not unrealistic to lose 5 pounds a week. So in just a month you can be 20 pounds lighter.

3. Reward Yourself

If any of you have ever trained a dog you know how important rewards are. They're important to you too so be sure to set some. For example, if I lose 20 pounds in two months I will treat myself to a meal at my favorite restaurant.

4. Bet with Yourself

The more extreme you make the bet, the more you have to lose. Go to a friend and tell them, "If I don't lose 20 pounds in the next two months I'll walk your dog for a month." If you want to motivate yourself even more "Go to your boss and tell him if you don't lose 20 pounds in the next two months you'll work for free for two weeks.

There are four great ways to motivate yourself to get the job done. You can lose that extra weight and you can do it fast.

The Relationship between Weight and Emotions

Believe it or not, your emotions play a vital role in your weight condition. Sometimes, depressed people prefer to eat more food to relieve their discomfort feeling. Others also turn to food for comfort, especially when they are stressed and frustrated from their work. As a result, this action may lead to weight gain. It is said that the more you understand about how emotions affect your eating habits, the better prepared you will be to overcome some hindrances that occur to control your daily food consumption.

Emotional eating refers to the act of eating to feel better. Most people see food as more than a source of body energy. Sometimes, they enjoy eating, especially during their leisure time. There is nothing wrong with this habit. However, you should always know your limitations when it comes to food intake.

People often eat to deal with their bad feelings. But, this habit may lead to severe eating disorders, depression, obesity and weight gain. If you don't want to experience any health issues because of excessive intake of foods, you need to find ways of how to solve this problem.

Tips on How to Fight Emotional Eating

Some people find it hard to handle their emotions and eating habits. If you are one of them, you should always know the different strategies to manage your weight. For your guide, here they are:

• Rate Your Hunger Level – Before you start eating, rate your hungry level. From 1 to 10, ten scales are the highest and it means that you are full. If you realize that your hunger level is between 3 and 10, you need to avoid eating. You can only consume enough food if your hunger level is at 1 or 2 levels.

• Deal with Other Comforting Activities – Instead of eating more foods while you're stressed, try to search for any alternative activities that can alleviate your present condition. The typical examples of these are listening to your favorite music, playing a musical instrument, chatting with your friends or going for a walk.

• Practice Daily Exercise – It is undeniable that regular training can help in reducing weight. But, it can also help in dealing with anxiety and stress. Through daily exercise, you can prevent from over eating. Therefore, you can easily manage your emotions while developing your health condition.

• Use the Three Food Interference - This scheme is done through eating three kinds of nutritious foods first before eating your favorite foods. The typical healthy foods are vegetables, yogurt, fruits and many more.

As you can see, there are several ways to manage your emotions. Whether you are depressed or suffering from any emotional issues, you don't need to eat over and over again. Once you know how to handle your emotions, you are not tempted to eat more food.

Chapter 6- Why You Should Not Skip Exercise

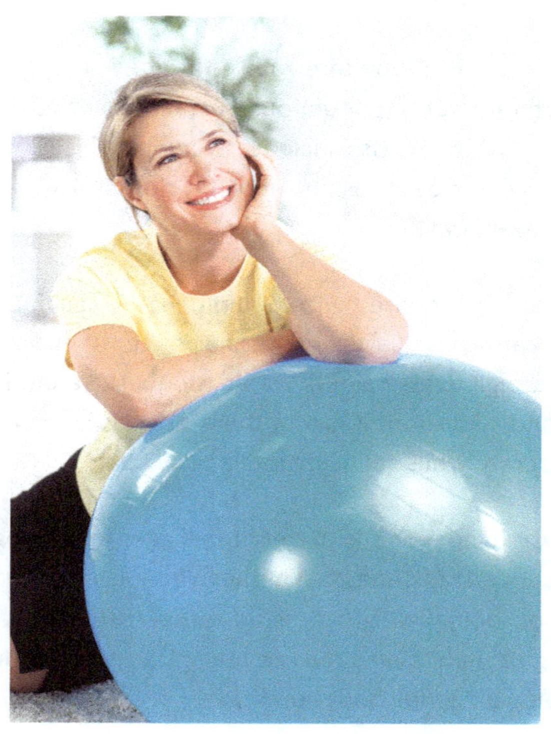

Exercise and weight loss revolves around a single word – calories. Though people need food to survive, there is always a limitation. Say for instance, excessive consumption of carbohydrates is not advisable. To burn more fats, you need to practice a couple of exercises. Whether you want a mild or intense routine, you should always follow its procedures.

An ideal exercise for weight loss includes a combination of weight training and aerobic exercises. Experts claim that if a person keeps on performing daily exercises, they have a better chance of keeping the weight off longer and achieving a healthier body condition.

Drop Those Fats, Tone Those Muscles

Since there are several exercises for weight loss, some of you may find it hard to pick one. To solve this issue, here are the few top training methods you should follow:

- Aerobics — This is a type of exercise that develops the breathing and heart rate for a continuous sustained period. The typical examples of this exercise include swimming, bicycling, stepping and walking. For best results, you can do at least two to three exercises every day.

- Cardiovascular Exercises with Equipment — Machines can offer multiple cardiovascular exercises. The common examples of these are elliptical trainers, stair climbers, adaptive motion trainers and a lot more. Most of these devices help in monitoring your heart rate while reducing more body fats.

- Strength Training — This is perfect to all ages and recognized as a vital component of fitness. Whether you wish to practice lifting weights or doing weight-resistance exercises, it can help in increasing or maintaining muscle mass. It can also reduce weight and develop a healthy body condition.

Aside from the above mentioned, there are several exercises for weight loss. In fact, there are some people who prefer to enter in several fitness gyms. For those who are quite busy, they prefer to perform intense exercises at home.

As you keep on exercising, your heart rate tends to increase. As a result, your metabolism also develops and chances to burn more fats are largely increase. For every minute of training, you can burn a specific amount of calories. The burned calories depend on how dynamic the exercise is you are performing. Studies have shown that the more calories you burn during exercises, the more calories you deficit. Therefore, you can lose more weight within a short period of time.

In addition, when you continue doing the training, glucose is slowly depleted. Then, the body turns to its fat storage and burns the inner fat to make energy in replacement of the glucose. It means that when you burn fatter, losing weight will be noticeable.

Even if there are multiple exercises for weight loss, some still find it hard to achieve their ultimate goal. If you are one of them, the best option that you should take is to make a journal. In your journal, you have to write down your daily activity. You also need to itemize the different meals that you need to consume while doing the training. To ensure that you will follow your training plan, you have to encourage yourself. You can also list down your multiple reasons why you opt to lose weight. That way you are always inspired to perform the needed activities.

The First is Cardio Training

The topic of losing weight can often elicit "groans." There's no need you know. In fact, did you know that cardio training can lead to quickly building muscle mass and losing weight? Cardio training can be as simple or as complex as you like. Walking, jogging, and cycling are all goof forms of aerobic exercise that can quickly burn body fat. Aerobic exercises are a great choice for the entire body.

There's all kinds of sites promoting the "secret to successful weight loss" online but it's really not as complicated as we might want to make it out to be. If you want to lose weight quickly then you must change the ration between calorie intake and calorie use. You can either increase your exercise or decrease your calories. The best plan of attack is to combine the two. Reduce your calories by no more than 500 and increase your activity with a daily 30 minutes of cardio a day.

When you build muscle you burn fat. Strength training builds muscle. Squats, lunges, and pushups require no equipment and are very effective. Free weights are also very effective – dumbbells can be purchased for cheap and cans always work too. Don't make this more expensive or complicated than it has to be.

Fat burning aerobic exercise is different than recreational exercise. For example Tennis and golf are recreational exercise and won't do a thing for your weight loss, or very little. Aerobic exercise like running, walking, and jogging even for just 30 minutes will get the heart pumping and the fat melting.

For a while it was thought that low intensity exercises would do the job of burning fat but that myth was quickly dismissed. If you don't get your heart rate up you won't burn fat. When you have a high intensity aerobic workout you will consume around 70% of the body's energy. This means calories are burnt and that includes fat cells.

Your cardio workout can be as little as 10 to 15 minutes but a 45 to 60 minute workout is the most effective for burning fat. Don't think for a minute that more is better, because after 60 minutes the amount of weight loss actually goes down not up.

Cardio training can lose weight and build muscles quickly but when it comes to healthy weight loss that you can maintain you'll want to ensure you have a healthy lifestyle.

Kimberly Jackson
Muscle Building Always Feel Great!

Whether this is the first time you've decided to lose weight or your hundredth attempt you can do this. You can build muscle, lose fat fast, and feel great. So how do you go about doing this? Glad you asked!

It all begins with building muscle. Now don't worry you're not going to turn yourself into the incredible hulk. Women in particular worry that they'll become too muscular and that just doesn't happen without some very specialized work.

As you build muscle, your weight may actually increase. Don't worry; this is okay, because muscle actually weighs more than fat. As your muscles develop, your body will begin to burn fat faster. Your weight training is really quite simple — squats, pushups, and free weights are all the equipment you need.

You're going to that weight training with cardio exercises to burn fat. Either 30 minutes a day or two 15 minute sessions will be enough cardio to enjoy the benefits. Cardio is as simple as a brisk walk. Of course, there are all kinds of cardio exercises including jogging, cycling, circuit training, and tons of other excellent aerobic exercises. A treadmill can be a great investment because of the convenience of that walk indoors no matter what the weather. Your cardio should raise your heart rate but not make you out of breath.

You will also need to look at your diet. To build muscle you need to make sure you are taking 25% to 30% of your calories in protein. You'll want to avoid fats, and add plenty of fiber to your diet. Fiber is filling and so you'll eat less. Avoid eating all processed and packaged foods, which contain little nutrition. Instead, stick to fresh fruits and vegetables, poultry, fish, and lean meat cuts.

Drop Those Fats, Tone Those Muscles

For many of us, belly fat is our biggest enemy. It's also the hardest to lose. Don't make the mistake of thinking that as long as you do hundreds of crunches will do the job. All that will happen is the muscle under the fat will develop and your belly will look larger. Cardio exercises are needed to burn belly fat!

Great, we've covered how to build muscle and lose fat fast, but there's more to it than exercise and caloric intake. One of the biggest reasons why weight loss fails is failing to have a plan, so get your plan in place. Finally, don't wait to get motivated. Set goals, reward yourself, get up, and get moving. Before you know it, you'll have shed those extra pounds.

CHAPTER 7- THE BASICS OF WEIGHT MAINTENANCE

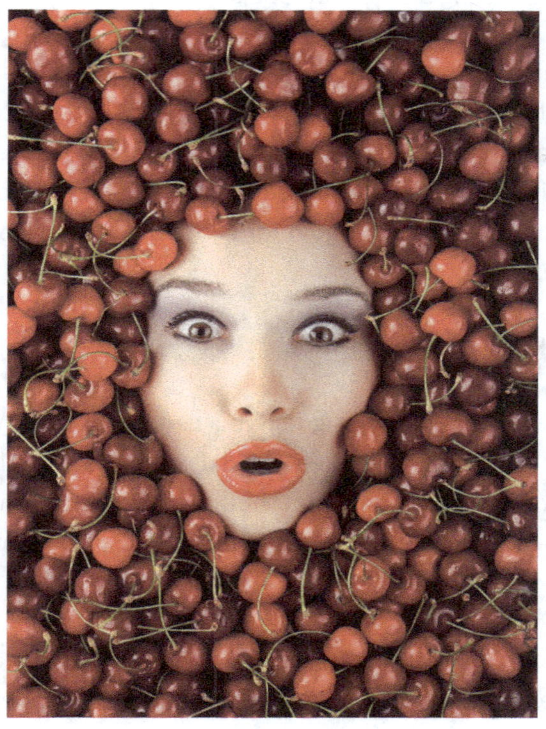

If you wish to lose weight, you need to set up your ultimate goal. You also need to achieve your goals no matter what it takes. It says that setting realistic goals before you start a weight loss plan is proven effective.

Sometimes, people find it hard to set up weight loss and maintenance goals. Instead of worrying about this issue, accurate research is an ideal option. You can also seek help from experts and trusted friends for wide details.

The accurate steps in setting up weight loss goals are not too complicated. Whether you are a beginner or not, you can easily make your own plan. For more details, here are some steps you should know:

Step 1: Start Setting Small Daily Goals

Before aiming to lose more pounds of weight, your first goal is to reduce at least one pound every week. This is easier to achieve than reducing more weight in an instant. To ensure that you achieve this goal, you have to set your mind state. You need to remind yourself about your goal for continuous daily workouts and healthy lifestyle.

Step 2: Make Advanced Goals

Once you achieve your first goal, you need to level it up. Say for instance, if you already reached the daily 30-minute walk goal, you need to extend it to a daily one-hour walk. You also need to eat smaller portions every meal. For best results, you have to seek counseling from experts.

Step 3: Know Your Ultimate Goal – If you wish to have a perfect body figure and weight, you need to make ways to achieve it. Aside from daily routines, you need to learn how to cook healthy foods, engage in fitness programs and other related activities.

Step 4: Organize Time Frames for Your Goals

If you notice that you are continuously reaching for your ultimate goals, you have to reward yourself. Depending on your preferences, you can go shopping, take a weekend trip, and get a facial and a lot more.

Though you already reached your main goal, you have to practice daily exercise and a healthy lifestyle. This can help in maintaining your body and weight the way you want it to be.

While setting up weight loss and maintenance goals, you should always be realistic. This means that you don't need to jot down just any activities, especially when you can't really achieve them. During your first week of the weight loss program, make sure that you can do it and you have ample time to perform any related exercises.

Significance of Setting Weight Loss and Maintenance Goals

If you know how to set up weight loss and maintenance goals, you don't have to worry about your daily activities. Since you need to jot down all the activities that you need to do, you are always guided on how to reduce more weight.

Through finalizing your exact goals, you don't need to ask your friends or other experts on what objective it is that you really want to achieve. Therefore, it is easy for you to find ways to reach your preferred goals.

How to Eat Right

Eating right doesn't mean that you need to follow strict dietary plans. If you wish to eat the right amount and types of food, all you need to do is to know the different foods that are loaded with perfect nutrients. You can do this through asking assistance from experts or by reading health books.

Drop Those Fats, Tone Those Muscles

If you wish to lose weight, you need to focus on your daily meals. You have to know not only the foods that you need to eat, but also the foods that can trigger your weight condition. Instead of worrying about this issue, here are some tips you should consider:

• Know the Exact Foods You Need to Consume

Some people restrain themselves from eating to reduce weight. This scheme is not advisable. If you are hungry, then, you need to eat but with limitations. If you keep on eating fewer amounts of food, you might suffer from complicated health problems like fatigue.

• Consume More Fresh Vegetables and Fruits

Nutritious foods can help you lose weight. These foods are perfect instead of consuming unhealthy meals every day. If you switch into a healthy lifestyle, expect that you will lose weight and have a perfect body condition.

• Avoid Skipping Meals

If you keep on skipping meals, you may become hungrier for the next meal. As much as possible, you need to eat five to six times a day. But, you have to eat a small amount. Never multi-task and don't watch television while eating. While eating, just sit and pay attention to your food.

• Drink More Water

Your body needs more water. Drinking more water is highly recommended than consuming soda drinks. Before eating, you have to drink some water to reduce your food intake. This can help in reducing more body fat.

• Make a Journal

Making a journal is an effective way to monitor your daily eating habits. Depending on your preferred meals, you need to jot it down and you will know the exact amount of food you intake.

• Try New Foods

Even if you are planning to lose weight, it doesn't mean that you need to deprive yourself from eating your favorite foods. Instead of eating the same types of food over and over again, you need to try new and healthy recipes.

• Clean Your Kitchen

It means that you need to remove all food that can destroy your regular healthy diet. As much as possible, buy only some food that is suggested by your nutritionist. This is an excellent move to refrain you from eating your favorite chips or other unhealthy foods.

Through your knowledge on how to eat right, you don't have to worry about your weight and body condition. You can easily motivate yourself to reduce more fat. If you are still confused on how to eat right, you are free to consult your nutritionist.

Take note that there is nothing wrong with you eating food. Just make sure that you are eating the right and healthy ones. You also need to monitor your daily intake to avoid weight gain. If you are motivated and committed to your specific goal, you can achieve it no matter what it takes.

The truth is we can build muscle and lose weight fast. Failure often comes on the hands of poor information. There are 5 common myths about fast weight loss that you shouldn't believe.

Myth #1 – I overeat so there's no way I'll ever lose fat quickly.

Overeating is mostly the result of stress – when a person is worried, depressed, scared, sad, or anxious overeating is often the result. Decrease your stress and you'll be surprised at how fast you lose pound. Becoming physically active can lead to a loss in weight.

Myth #2 – My genetics mean I'll always be overweight.

Being fat isn't a result of your genetics. Yes some families may have a pattern of being overweight but you can overcome your genes and lose fat quickly. Your genetics don't control your weight, your lifestyle choices do. Watch a couple of episodes of "The Biggest Loser" if you want proof.

Myth #3 – I'm fat because of a slow metabolism.

It's true that when your thyroid isn't functioning properly it can slow your metabolism and bring your fat loss to a halt. However most people that believe they have a slow metabolism really don't. Instead what they have is a need to jumpstart the body with a combination of good nutrition and aerobic exercise. It's a simple as a 15 minute brisk walk.

Myth #4 – It's possible to keep the weight off even with a fad diet.

If you want to quickly lose 10 pounds a fad diet will certainly allow you to accomplish that quickly. But the research indicates that 80%

of dieters will actually gain the weight back in 5 years. Worse, you'll also lose muscle mass and gain back fat. This might explain why society seems to be getting more overweight as the years go by.

Losing the weight using a diet (even a fad diet) isn't so bad as long as you follow up with healthy lifestyle changes that ensure you keep the weight off.

Myth #5 – I can lose my belly fat doing crunches

Far too many people attempt to get rid of belly fat with no success. What happens is muscle builds under the belly fat and then your belly actually looks bigger. If you want to lose belly fat faster aerobic exercise is the answer – in fact, you'll lose belly fat as much as 10x faster with cardiac exercises.

Now that we've uncovered these 5 myths you'll be shedding those extra pounds faster than ever.

CHAPTER 8- OF PILLS AND SURGERIES

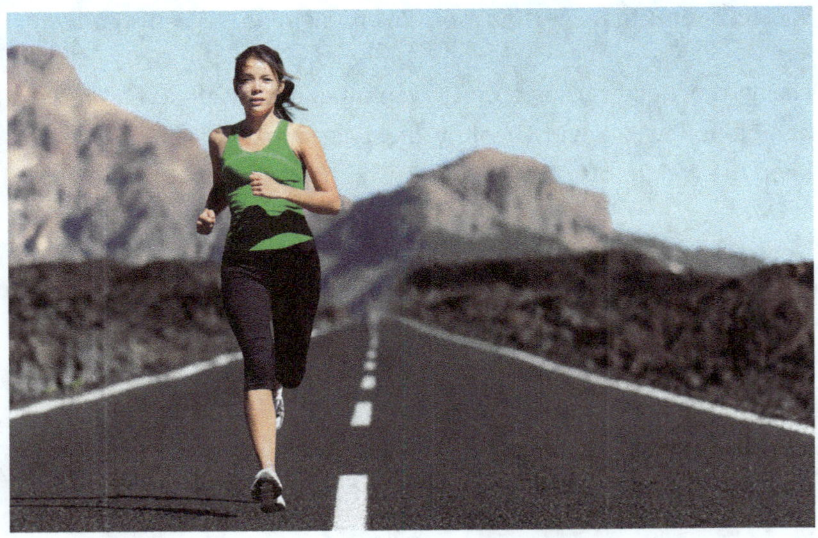

To lose weight, some people prefer to purchase supplements or pills. Others also desire to undergo several surgical procedures. Whatever options you will take, you have to be more knowledgeable on how they work.

If you wish to depend on pills to lose weight, you need to examine each supplement available on the market. In some cases, people prefer to get expensive pills thinking that they are more effective compared to cheap ones. Whether you pick affordable or expensive types, you can't easily determine its exact function if you don't understand its various ingredients.

Before buying any pills or supplements, the best option that you should take is to start reading its reviews. While reading reviews, you have to browse not only one but various websites. The more reviews you read, the more chances of getting more valuable information you have. To ensure that you get an ideal type of pill for weight loss, it is best to seek help from experts. You can also ask your doctors about the exact brand and type of pill that you need to take.

Since money plays a vital role in buying effective pills for weight loss, you don't need to depend on a very expensive one. In fact, there are several pills or supplements that are cheap but come with effective results. Just make sure that you compare one pill to another for perfect buying.

Whether you want to buy pills through local or online schemes, make sure that you examine your preferred shop. Some shops are effective while others are not. To ensure that you will never be deceived by any scam supplier, always read the different testimonials of their previous and current customers. This can help you in deciding if your desired shop is offering an ideal supplement or not.

Are Surgeries Effective in Losing Weight?

For those who can afford it, they prefer to depend on surgical procedures to remove their excessive body fat. If you are one of them, you have to find the best surgeon. Searching for the best surgeon is not too difficult. You can find one through asking assistance from your trusted friends. You can also read some reviews online to get a reliable surgeon.

Surgical procedures for losing weight are also effective. However, you have to follow the prescriptions of your surgeon before and after the surgery. You also need to be more conscious with your daily activities to avoid any side effects.

Whether you wish to undergo surgical procedures, take pills or practice the natural way of losing weight, you can get your preferred results. Just make sure that you know how to do it accurately to ensure positive outcomes.

Creating Body Image Goals

Lasting relationship are achievable as long as you preserve your beauty in and out. As some advice, it is good to have an inspiration and motivation to conduct this particular healthy act of living. You can look for reasons like work, family, and love life and even friend and relationship concerns. It is a common fact that people will only accept you based on their first impression, and it is true that they cannot appreciate you as a person at a first glance. This is just a sample of motivation that you can use for you to immediately realize the importance of body image for the public's eyes.

Work habits need a lot of effort and energy execution. This reason can be used as a motivation for you to pursue living healthier while having a good body. As long as you exercise and eat appropriate types of food, you can generate positive system for your body such as intelligence and energy. As a result, you will no longer have to worry about the outcomes and accomplishments that will soon happen after you perform your job efficiently and effectively accompanied with a suitable amount of push and motivations.

Relationship will never have a good foundation if both partners do not possess the motivation to become a good person in relation to inside and outside appearance. It is better to be aware of how you can make yourself a good person and that it will also reflect on how you appear from the outside. Body image can also be one of the greatest motivations for a relationship to become stronger in terms of foundation. Yes love is more important, but maintaining a considerable appearance can generate more passion in love. As a matter of fact, body image can be more beneficial because it can make people that are in a relationship be in a more passionate state of romance when making love which is very healthy for love, connection, and communication.

Your family, especially your children, need your time and effort when the day ends after long and busy working hours. In this case, it is a motivation for you to become more energetic because your work is not the only entity that needs your full attention. It is better to patronize healthy living by means of exercising to promote the beneficial effects for your family that can only possibly delivered by a good image of body.

CHAPTER 9- 10 SUPER FOODS TO MUSCLE BUILDING

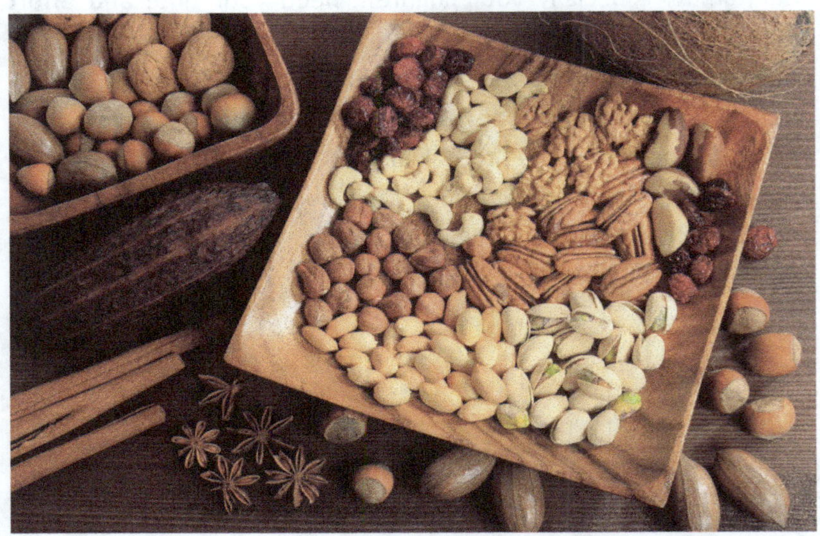

In order to build muscle and lose weight you need a variety of veggies, carbs, fruits, proteins, and healthy fats. In order to quickly build muscle and lose weight you need 10 super foods.

1. Whole Eggs – Eggs are one of the cheapest super foods offering you an excellent source of protein. The cholesterol that we hear so much about isn't a problem. If you have cholesterol problems lower your body fat not the eggs you consume.

2. Flax Seeds – Here's an excellent source of fiber, omega 3, and protein. Grind the flax seeds and sprinkle on your berries or yogurt. Don't use flax oil as it's unstable and has no fiber benefits

3. Quinoa – In South America Quinoa is considered the king of grains. The fiber and protein in Quinoa is higher than that in oats and rice, plus its gluten free.

4. Mixed Nuts – Nuts are packed with mono and polyunsaturated fats, fiber, proteins, Vitamin e, potassium, zinc, and magnesium. Nuts are dense in calories so if you are skinny and looking to put on a few pounds these will do it.

5. Wild Salmon – Omega 3 fatty acids are found in salmon, as well as providing 20 grams of protein per 100 gram serving.

6. Fish Oil – Taking fish oil can reduce inflammation in the body, increase testosterone levels, and lower body fat. Take 900mg per day. It's hard to get this level eating fish.

7. Berries – Fresh berries are a powerful antioxidant keeping you healthy and helping you to improve your weight loss.

8. Green Tea – Another strong antioxidant and a powerful natural diuretic. It can speed up fat loss, improve blood sugar, and prevent cancer.

9. Water – Something as simple water is considered a super food and vital to your weight loss program, muscle development, and health. You should drink at least 8 glasses a day.

10. Tomatoes – High in lycopene they are an excellent cancer preventer and a benefit in your strength training. You can't eat too many tomatoes!

These 10 super foods combined with an overall healthy diet, a cardiac workout, and some strength training and in no time you'll be pounds lighter. Super foods can help you to quickly build muscles and lose weight. Being overweight is hazardous to your health and to your self-esteem. Why not set your goals and get motivated? You'll be feeling better about your weight in no time at all.

11. Acai berry - The buzz of Acai Berry seems to have traveled quickly around the globe. This is one of the best antioxidant foods out there and the Acai Berry Select Weight Loss Supplement has been talked about by Dr. Oz as being a successful tool by many.

Other Helpful Food Tips

1. Watch what you eat – You should be keeping an eye on everything you put in your mouth. It's the garnishes, and the extras that can be packed with calories.

2. Fried foods are bad – If you want to lose weight fast, you need to avoid fried foods completely. Even if you drain or soak off the oil, it's within the food. To lose weight quickly take fried food out of your diet.

3. Only fresh fruit juice – We all know how important it is to drink plenty of water but sometimes we have a craving for something other than water. In that case, you should choose fresh fruit juice that contains no added sweeteners, which translate to calories.

4. Go vegetable crazy – When it comes to weight loss vegetables are your best choice. While all veggies are good for you, leafy greens are your best choice. Make sure you include them in your salad. Fresh veggies contain the nutrients you need and they offer important fiber to the diet. They make great snack foods and can quickly take care of hunger pangs.

5. No between-meal snacks –This is a common problem for people on the move. They get hungry and grab whatever junk food is nearest to take away the hunger pains. These are not only calories you don't need or want; there is also a great deal of fat in these snack foods. Just eliminating junk food snacks and soda can easily

lead to a 2 to 3 pound reduction a month, without doing anything else.

6. Your diet should be made up of 30% protein – If you are going to build muscle, you need protein. Muscle burns fat and so you've got a winning situation here.

ABOUT THE AUTHOR

Kimberly Jackson was born in Minnesota but grew up in Pennsylvania. She was the third in a five sisters, two of whom struggled with obesity at an early age. Her father also died because of a common obesity complication – heart attack.

Her experiences molded Kimberly's desire to educate all those who would listen about the harmful effects of storing too much body fat. She built her gym out of this desire.

Today, Kimberly is a mother of two. She remains to be very active in her campaign for weight and good nutrition.

www.ingramcontent.com/pod-product-compliance
Lightning Source LLC
Chambersburg PA
CBHW070050260726
48658CB00002B/829